THE KETO COOKBOOK

Simple and Healthy Keto Diet Recipes
including 10 Ultimate Weight Loss Tips

2nd Edition

Kylie Reid

TABLE OF CONTENTS

Introduction 1

Details On the Keto Diet? 3
    What's This I Heard About the Keto Flu? 4
    History of the Keto Diet 5
    Basics of the Keto Diet 6

Advantages of a Keto Diet 7
    You'll Lose Abdominal Fat 8
    Your Blood Sugar and Insulin Levels Will Improve 9
    It Positively Affects Your Cholesterol 10
    You'll Feel Less Hungry 11

Which Foods Can I Eat and What is Prohibited? 13
    What You Can Eat 13
        Meats 13
        Dairy that's High in Fat 14
        Seafood 14
        Berries 14
        Vegetables 14
        Seasonings 15
        Oils and Fats 15
        Nuts 15
        Beverages 15
    Is Prohibited 16
        Processed Foods 16
        Grains 16
        Root Vegetables 16
        Legumes 16
        Sweets 17
        Alcohol 17

Sauces 17

How Do I Prepare for my Keto Diet? 19

One Week Before 20

Three to Four Days Before 20

One to Two Days Before 21

Recipes For Breakfast 23

Jalapeno and Cheese Egg Cups 24

Breakfast Roll Ups 25

Keto Porridge 26

Keto Mashed Cauliflower and Bacon Patties 27

Ham and Spinach Casserole 28

Cheese Waffles 29

Eggs and Bacon 30

Ham and Spinach Frittata 32

Mayonnaise and Boiled Eggs 33

Hardboiled Eggs With Bacon and Avocado 34

Scrambled Eggs with Cheese 36

Cauliflower Hash Browns 37

Tuna Salad And Hot Peppers 38

Scrambled Eggs Mexican-Style 39

Keto Friendly Pancakes 41

Recipes for Lunch 43

Egg Salad 44

Zucchini and Sausage Boats 45

Meatless Keto Club Salad 46

Eggplant and Cheese Keto "Bread" 48

Mushroom and Cauliflower Grits 49

Keto Caprese Salad 51

Keto Taco Salad 52

Avocado and Chicken Salad 53

Egg Salad with Avocado 54

Chili 55

Beef Stew 56

Lettuce Wrapped Cheeseburgers 57

Healthy Green Smoothie 59

Keto-Friendly Chicken Sandwich 60

Crock Pot Pizza 61

Recipes for Dinner 63

Skillet Enchilada Chicken 64

Zucchini with Walnut Pesto 65

Cauliflower Salad 67

Keto Spinach and Watercress Salad 68

Zucchini Nests 69

Keto Cheeseburger and Bacon Casserole 70

Garlic Seasoned Scallops 71

Salmon With Miso 72

Lemon Fish Fillets 73

Keto Tuna Casserole 74

Stuffed Beef Rolls 76

Shrimp Alfredo 78

Taco Soup 79

Oven Baked Pork Chops with Salad 80

Keto Meatloaf 81

Recipes for Snacks and Desserts 83

Macadamia Nut Fat Bombs 84

Keto Zucchini Bread 85

Matcha Cheesecake 87

Flourless Brownies 88

Coconut Chip Cookies 89

Peanut Butter and Coconut Balls 90

Sugarless Cheesecake 91

Coconut Ice Cream 93

Raspberry and Vanilla Keto Smoothie 94

Pecan and Chocolate Bark 95

Bonus! 10 Keto Diet Tips 97

Disclaimer 101

Imprint 102

Introduction

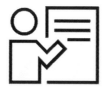

How much do you know about the Keto diet? It's much more than just a fad. In fact, the Keto diet has been around for centuries – since the time of the early Greeks. They realized that their gladiators became stronger when they followed a diet that was very low in carbs and high in healthy fats and proteins. Although the Keto diet was forgotten about for centuries after that, it has now become quite popular again, both with body builders and with those who want to lose weight.

Before you start following the Keto diet, read over the information provided below and scroll through the recipes. You'll find that it's very easy to follow and contain plenty of nutritional information. With them, you'll be able to follow this diet fairly easily.

Details On the Keto Diet?

Understanding the Keto Diet begins with a basic understanding of its name. "Keto" is short for "ketosis." When you follow a diet that's high in proteins and healthy fats, while at the same time, limiting the amount of carbohydrates or "carbs" that you eat, your body ends up going into a state of ketosis.

Ketosis is the name for when the fat stores in your body begin to be burned off in order to provide energy. These fat stores are in your liver as well, and they'll also disappear when you're in ketosis. You want this fat to disappear, because it will help you lose weight and give you additional energy.

There are many questions that arise when someone first considers following the Keto diet. They range from what foods you can eat to whether or not the Keto flu is real. Some of these questions are answered below.

The Keto flu is a real phenomenon, although not everyone who goes on this diet ends up with it. The most important thing to remember is that the keto flu isn't a real flu at all. Instead, it feels like you have the flu, since you'll feel achy and lethargic, but you won't have the sniffles or any of the other symptoms of the traditional flu.

This condition strikes many people within a few days of drastically cutting back on carbohydrates. In fact, it's a direct reaction to this. Your body needs to adjust to your new diet, and this is exactly how that happens. The lack of carbs and beginnings of ketosis send your system into shock, and you'll end up feeling low on energy and pretty cruddy for a day or so. It's a sign that the diet is working.

With that said, you can manage your symptoms so that you don't end up suffering from the Keto flu for more than a day or so, if it even strikes altogether. Some people, particularly those who ate few carbs to begin with, don't end up with the Keto flu. If you are one of the unlucky ones, the best way of dealing with it is just to power through. Drink some unsweetened coffee to help with the brain fog and lethargy, take an over the counter painkiller to counteract the aches and pains, and then keep moving. Before you know it, you'll feel better again and the you'll be on your way to ketosis and weight loss.

Some of the history of the Keto diet has already been mentioned. It started with the Ancient Greeks, but then it vanished for several thousand years. The diet reappeared in the 1920s when several scientists decided to test it on people with epilepsy. At the time, there weren't any good medications for the condition. Those that did exist had very unpleasant side effects and they didn't work as well as the ones that we have today. The scientists put several patients with epilepsy on a low carbohydrate, high protein diet, and observed how many seizures they had over the course of several weeks. As it turns out, the diet drastically lessened the amount of seizures that they had. The Keto diet became a good option for people with epilepsy.

Jumping ahead more than a few decades, the diet emerged into the mainstream back in the 1980s. At that point, it was very popular with body builders who realized that it allowed them to lose fat while gaining muscle at the same time. However, it wasn't until the 1990s when the Keto diet really began to take off. This is due to the parents of a child named Charlie Abrams. Charlie had a very severe form of epilepsy and after trying numerous medications without much luck, his father, Tim, put him on the Keto diet. Charlie had some immediate health changes thanks to the diet and began to improve. He was featured on an episode the television show *Dateline* back in 1994. This brought the diet into the mainstream. It became very popular and turned from a specialized diet for people with epilepsy and for bodybuilders into one that's a good way to lose weight in general.

BASICS OF THE KETO DIET

In order to follow the Keto diet, you need to count your macros and micros. These are methods of measuring the nutrition that you receive each day. Macros are things like protein, carbohydrates, and fat. They are what your body needs in order to keep running. Micros, on the other hand, consist of the smaller nutrients. Things like Vitamin A, Vitamin C, and Vitamin B, as well as Potassium, Magnesium, and more are all micros.

People on the Keto diet need to measure the amounts of their macros and micros for several reasons. First, you must not eat too many carbs, lest your body go out of ketosis. Secondly, you need to keep your fat and protein counts at the right numbers in order to remain healthy. The micros play a large part in this as well.

Now that you know what the Keto diet involves and how you can follow it, it's time to go into a bit more depth. We'll start with the many advantages to being on this diet.

Advantages of a Keto Diet

There are several important advantages of following the Keto diet. We've already established that the diet is good for people with epilepsy, as it will help lower the overall number of seizures that suffers are known to have. It's also a good way to gain muscle mass, which is why body builders prefer it. The diet also gives people more energy and increased brain clarity. In addition, some of the many great benefits to this diet are:

YOU'LL LOSE ABDOMINAL FAT

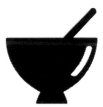

Unlike other diets, the Keto diet directly affects your abdominal fat. This means that you'll lose the weight in this area. With those other diets, you don't really have any control over where the weight comes off. For example, if you do a simple combination of eating less and exercising, women will lose weight in their chests and hips first. That stubborn abdominal fat may stick around. However, with the Keto diet, all of the fat cells in your abdomen will start to be burned off as soon as you reach ketosis. That fat is then used as energy. Essentially, you're able to control where you lose the weight.

YOUR BLOOD SUGAR AND INSULIN LEVELS WILL IMPROVE

People who are overweight tend to end up with blood sugar and insulin issues. This is why those who are obese almost always get diagnosed with diabetes. The excess abdominal fat makes it hard for the pancreas to work properly, which means that you'll end up with high blood sugar. When you're on the Keto diet and end up in a state of ketosis, you'll end up losing that problematic abdominal fat, which makes your pancreas work better. Plus, this diet is low in sugar and carbs, both of which are processed by the pancreas as well. Giving this organ a bit of a break makes it work better, and you'll see your blood sugar and insulin levels improve back to their normal, healthy state.

IT POSITIVELY AFFECTS YOUR CHOLESTEROL

Did you know that there are two main types of cholesterol? Your body produces both HDL and LDL cholesterol. One is the "good" kind. You want that number to be high. A larger amount of good cholesterol in your body can counteract the bad, making it less likely that you'll end up with heart disease. There's also LDL, or "bad" cholesterol. The higher this number, the more likely you are to have a heart attack or a stroke. You need this number to be in the appropriately low range. When you start to cut back on the amount of carbs that you eat when you're on the Keto diet, your LDL numbers will decrease while the HDL ones rise, making your cardiovascular system much healthier.

YOU'LL FEEL LESS HUNGRY

On top of all of the other advantages described here, following the Keto diet means that you'll be less hungry. Many people don't realize this, but the amount of carbs that they eat actually makes them hungry. They fuel other sugar cravings, making you hungrier for more carbs. As a result, you end up trapped in a vicious cycle. The Keto diet breaks this cycle, and followers feel full longer, so they snack less.

Which Foods Can I Eat and What is Prohibited?

The goal of the Keto diet is to move you into ketosis andthen stay there. This means that you need to eat a diet that's very low in carbs and sugar, while remaining high in protein and healthy fats. When you're on the Keto diet, you need to eat certain foods on a regular basis, while avoiding others. Here's a quick breakdown of your options:

WHAT YOU CAN EAT

Meats

Meat is one of the main staples of the Keto diet. This means that you can eat more than one type while on the Keto diet. They include: steak, lamb, ground beef, chicken, turkey, pork, bacon (in limited amounts, since bacon tends to be very fatty), sausage, ham, and more.

Dairy that's High in Fat

While you'll need to avoid some types of dairy, you can eat high fat options, like sour cream, cream cheese, heavy whipping cream, and cheese in general.Cottage cheese and plain yogurt are on the list. Eggs are also allowed.

Seafood

Seafood is very good for you, as it contains a lot of protein and very little fat. Some of the best options are scallops, crab, mussels, clams, catfish, oysters, lobster, cod, tuna, and halibut. Really, any type of seafood can be eaten while on the Keto diet.

Berries

Going on the Keto diet doesn't mean that you're forever prohibited from eating sugar. It just means that you need to do so sparingly and stick with natural sugars. Some berries, like blueberries, blackberries, and strawberries, can be eaten in very small amounts.

Vegetables

You need to be careful when choosing which vegetables to include in your diet. Some contain hidden carbs and sugars. Your best options are olives, zucchini, green beans, broccoli, peppers, onions, spinach, and more. Basically, with the exception of eggplant, stick with green-colored vegetables.

Seasonings

Many different spices are on the list of foods that you can eat. They're necessary in order to make your food taste good.

Oils and Fats

You need to be able to cook your foods! This is why many oils and fats are allowed when you're on the Keto diet. Your options include things like butter, mayonnaise, coconut oil, olive oil, lard, avocado oil, and even ghee.

Nuts

Nuts are very high in protein, which makes them a great snack option for people on the Keto diet. Some of the very best ones to eat are walnuts, peanuts, almonds, pecans, hazelnuts, macadamia nuts, and butters made from either peanuts or almonds.

Beverages

Water isn't your only option when on the Keto diet. You can drink several different types of beverages, including black coffee, unsweetened tea, and alcoholic options like dry wine and hard liquor.

Processed Foods

Any foods that are premade and processed, such as boxed cereals and snack bars, even the ones that claim to be organic and low in calories, tend to contain a lot of carbohydrates and sugars.

Grains

Grains are full of carbohydrates and should be avoided when you're on the Keto diet. They include foods made with carbs as well, such as pizza, oatmeal, cereals, pasta, and granola. Other grains to avoid are corn and certain types of flours, including wheat, oats, quinoa, rye, millet, buckwheat, and more. Nut flours are allowed.

Root Vegetables

Root vegetables are very starchy and full of carbohydrates. You should take potatoes, carrots, rutabagas, yams, beets, parsnips, and turnips out of your diet.

Legumes

Many followers of the Keto diet claim that you can eat legumes, while others believe that they should be avoided entirely. To be on the safe side, you should eat lentils, chickpeas, kidney beans, navy beans, and more very sparingly, if at all.

Sweets

Candy, chocolate, cupcakes, cookies, and more are out, unless you make them yourself and know that they are Keto friendly, like the ones in our dessert section. You also need to steer clear of ice cream, various fruits (including watermelon, pineapple, peaches, plums, apples, limes, lemons, mango, cherries, grapes, bananas, and more), and custard and pudding.

Alcohol

Some types of alcohol are allowed (see the section above), but most should be avoided. This means that you shouldn't drink sweet wines, beer, mixed drinks or hard cider.

Sauces

Most sauces are tomato based and have additional sweeteners added in. This means that you can't have ketchup, mustard, barbecue sauce, or other options while on the diet.

How Do I Prepare for my Keto Diet?

A lot of the Preparation for the Keto diet is mental. You need to be mentally ready to cut back on the amount of carbs that you eat. Since many people eat a lot of carbohydrates on a daily basis, this is the biggest hurdle to jump over. Other methods of preparing for the diet involve stocking your kitchen with the right kind of foods. It all starts the week before you officially begin the diet.

ONE WEEK BEFORE

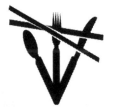

Approximately one week before you start the Keto diet, start cutting back on the number of carbohydrates that you eat. Each day, eat fewer of them. This will help you ease into the diet without shocking your system.

While you're doing this, begin planning out your meals. Go over the recipes in this cookbook and determine which of them you want to start with.

THREE TO FOUR DAYS BEFORE

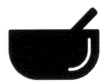

Several days before you start the diet, purge your kitchen and pantry of items that contain carbs. Go over the list above and give those items away (hint: if they are in unopened packaging, you can take them to your local foodbank). You need to get those carb-laden foods out of your house in order to avoid the temptation. Thankfully, once you've been on the diet for a bit, this feeling will fade and you won't want to wreck your progress.

ONE TO TWO DAYS BEFORE

At this point, it's time to head to the grocery store and begin stocking your pantry with Keto-friendly foods. Once your kitchen is ready and you're mentally prepared, you can start the diet!

Recipes For Breakfast

Jalapeno and Cheese Egg Cups

Time: 30 Minutes | Serves 6
Macros Per Serving: | Calories: 157.17 | Fats: 12.28g | Carbs: 1.35g | Protein: 9.75g

Ingredients

♦ 2 jalapeno peppers, diced small with the seeds removed

♦ 3 packages ofthe cheese of your choice

♦ 1 package of cream cheese

♦ 5 eggs

♦ 7 pieces of bacon

♦ ¼ tspgarlic powder

♦ ¼ tsponion powder

♦ Pepper

♦ Salt

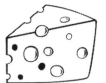

Preparation

1. Set the oven to 350 degrees F/190 degrees C

2. Throughly cook the bacon

3. Place the jalapenos, cheddar cheese, cream cheese, eggs, both seasonings and a little bit of the bacon grease in a bowl. Mix until blended. Season with pepper and salt.

4. Using a greased muffin pan, place a single bacon in each cup.

5. Add the uncooked egg mixture into each bacon-filled cup. The egg mixture should fill the cups halfway.

6. Bake the egg cups in the oven until they are done

Breakfast Roll Ups

Time: 20 Minutes | Serves 5
Macros: Calories: 412.2 | Fats: 31.66g | Carbs: 2.26g | Protein: 28.21g

Ingredients

♦ 1 ½ cups of shredded cheese

♦ 10 eggs

♦ ½ cup milk

♦ 5 slices of cooked bacon

♦ 5 cooked breakfast sausage patties

♦ Salt and pepper

Preparation

1. Crack the eggs over a bowl

2. Add water and then scramble the eggs, making sure to break the yolks

3. Pour some of the eggs into a pan that's been heated on the stove

4. Allow the eggs to cook until they are finished and then place two halves of one sausage patty and a single strip of bacon in the center

5. Sprinkle in cheese

6. Move the sides of the eggs to cover the fillings, it will be folded into thirds

7. Remove the breakfast roll from the pan

8. Repeat steps 1 through 7 until all five rolls ups have been made.

Keto Porridge

Time: 15 Minutes | Serves 1
Macros: Calories: 249 | Fats: 13.07g | Carbs: 5.78g | Protein: 17.82

Ingredients

- ◆ 4 tbsp flour made from coconuts
- ◆ 3 tsp protein powder, vanilla flavored
- ◆ 4 tsp meal, golden flaxseed
- ◆ 2 cups of milk, almond
- ◆ Powdered erythritol to taste
- ◆ Berries (if desired)

Preparation

1. Mix the coconut flour, vanilla protein powder, and golden flaxseed into a bowl and stir until completely together

2. Once mixed thoroughly, pour the grain mixture into a cooking pan, pour in the milk

3. Start heating it on low and then slowly raise it to hotter forms of heat, stirring as needed or occasionally until the mixture thickens and it's completely cooked

4. Add some erythritol on top if you wish.

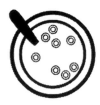

Keto Mashed Cauliflower and Bacon Patties

Time: 25 Minutes | Serves 3
Macros: Calories: 332.67 | Fats: 28.11g | Carbs: 8.6g | Protein: 10.65g

Ingredients

- 294 grams of cauliflower florets
- 3 tbsp whipping cream
- 6 tbsp of butter
- 3 sections of bacon
- ½ of an onion
- 50 grams of leeks
- 2 green onions
- 2 tsp garlic
- ½ cup of the cheese of your choice

Preparation

1. Put cauliflower, butter, and heavy whippingcream in a bowl that's a microwave-friendly

2. Microwave the mixture for five minutes, mix, and then microwave for another 4 minutes

3. Stir the entire mixture until it's creamy, and then add in the mozzarella cheese

4. Place the bacon in a pan and cook until it's thoroughly cooked, remove the bacon, but not the grease

5. Put the remaining Ingredients into a bowl and stir

6. Combine the bacon, garlic, onions, leeks, and cauliflower mixture together

7. Place more butter in a pan and melt it

8. Place three eggs rings in the warmed pan and pour the new mixture into each

9. Cook for several minutes on each side until it's done

Ham and Spinach Casserole

Time: 45 Minutes | Serves 15
Macros: Calories: 151.8 | Fats: 9.09g | Carbs: 1.35g | Protein: 15.1g

Ingredients

- 12 eggs
- 1/3 cup cream
- 1 cup of cheese, ricotta
- ½ onion
- ¼ tsp salt
- ½ tbsp garlic
- 2 cups of spinach
- 1 packaged of ham, diced

Preparation

1. Set the oven and preheat it to 350 degrees F/176 degrees C

2. Place the eggs in a bowl and scramble them

3. Add the cheese, and other Ingredients to the bowl and stir well

4. Fold the spinach and ham in the egg mixture bowl, making sure that they have plenty of eggs and seasoning on them

5. Add the entire mixture to a baking dish and then stir it together one more time

6. Bake for 40 minutes. Once the eggs are fully cooked they will puff slightly.

7. Top with some cheese (if you wish) before serving

Cheese Waffles

Time: 25 Minutes | Serves 12
Macros: Calories: 195.5 | Fats: 17.47g | Carbs: 3.49g | Protein: 5.49g

Ingredients

- 2 cups of flour, coconut
- 4 tsp of baking powder
- 2 tsp of sage, ground
- ¼ tsp onion powder
- ¼ tsp salt
- 3 cups milk, coconut
- Water
- 2 eggs
- 3 tsp coconut oil
- 1 cup cheese of your choice

Preparation

1. Turn on your waffle iron so that it can heat up

2. Mix salt, sage, coconut flour, baking powderand the garlic powder in a large bowl

3. Add the water, coconut milk, eggs, coconut oil and cheese into the bowlagain, stirring until they are well combined

4. Scoop a portion of the batter into your waffle iron, make as usual (note: the time to cook the waffles will depend on your waffle iron, some work at a hotter temperature than others)

Eggs and Bacon

Time: 20 Minutes | Serves 4
Macros: Calories: 272 | Fats: 22g | Carbs: 1g | Protein: 15g

Ingredients

♦ Package of sliced bacon

♦ 8 eggs

♦ Salt

♦ Pepper

♦ Parsley

♦ Spinach

♦ Tomatoes

Preparation

1. Place a frying pan on the stove and allow it to get hot. The pan will steam slightly

2. Carefully arrange each piece of the bacon on the pan in a thin layer (Note: you don't need to melt butter or use cooking oil when frying bacon.) Flip the bacon as you need to and cook it until it's very crispy and turning up at the edges.

3. Place the cooked bacon on several paper towels on a plate to drain some of the fat off of it.

4. Continue until you have cooked all of the bacon

5. Allow the panto cool and then remove some of the grease leaving just enough on to cook the eggs

6. Break the eggs over the pan one by one until the bottom of the pan has enough of them. Then add a bit of pepper and salt if you wish. When the whites around the yolk begin to harden, flip them with a spatula

7. Once the yolk is cooked enough for your taste, remove each egg and put them on a separate plate

8. Repeat until all of the eggs are cooked

9. Serve the bacon and eggs (top with a sprinkle of parsley)with some fresh spinach and a few tomatoes

Ham and Spinach Frittata

Time: 60 Minutes | Serves 4
Macros: Calories: 661 | Fats: 59g | Carbs: 4g | Protein: 27g

Ingredients

- 1 cup cubed ham
- 6 eggs
- 1/6 cup of water
- 1 cup of spinach
- 1 tbsp Butter
- Salt
- Pepper
- Cheese

Preparation

1. Place a frying pan on the stove and then heat it up. Once it's heated enough, put the ham into it.If you want, season the ham with some salt and pepper. Flip the ham over several times while it's cooking

2. Preheat the oven to 350 degrees F/176 degrees C

3. Set up a casserole dish by greasing the bottom

4. Crack the eggs into a bowl and begin to scramble them. Break the yolks and then mix thoroughly

5. Place the scrambled eggs in the casserole dish

6. Place the additional Ingredients into the dish and then gently stir them together

7. Place the casserole dish in the oven and then bake it for 45 minutes until everything is fully cooked. The top will feel a bit spongy

8. Remove the casserole dish. Allow it to cool for five minutes before serving

Mayonnaise and Boiled Eggs

Time: 20 Minutes | Serves 4
Macros: Calories: 316 | Fats: 29g | Carbs: 1g | Protein: 11g

Ingredients

- 5 eggs
- Water
- Salt
- Pepper
- Mayonnaise

Preparation

1. Place the eggs (shells and all) in a cooking pot

2. Place water in the pot until all of the eggs have water on them. They will float slightly. Put the pan on the stove and turn the heat on

3. Let the water boil and then set a cooking timer for ten minutes

4. Remove the eggs and set them aside to cool

5. Once the eggs have cooled, take their shells off of them. Cut them in half

6. Sprinkle a bit of salt and pepper on the eggs

7. Coat the eggs with some mayonnaise to taste

8. Serve the eggs

Hardboiled Eggs With Bacon and Avocado

Time: 20 Minutes | Serves 3
Macros: Calories: 144 | Fats: 13g | Carbs: 1g | Protein: 5g

Ingredients

♦ 4 slices of bacon

♦ 2 large eggs

♦ 1 ripe avocado

♦ Salt

♦ Pepper

Preparation

1. Place the eggs (shells and all) in a cooking pot

2. Add water to the pot until all of the eggs are covered and there is one inch of clearance (note: the eggs will float)

3. Place the pan on the stove and turn the heat onto high

4. Once the water boils, set a cooking timer for ten minutes

5. Place a frying pan on the stove over medium heat. Allow it to get hot. The pan will steam slightly

6. Carefully place each piece of bacon individually on the pan until the bottom of the pan is full. (Note: you don't need to melt butter or use cooking oil when frying bacon.) Flip the bacon as needed and cook until it is crispy and turning up at the edges.

7. Place the cooked bacon on several paper towels on a plate to drain some of the fat off of it. Once it has cooled, break the bacon into three to four pieces

8. Remove the eggs from the water and allow them to cool

9. Once the eggs have cooled, remove their shells and then slice in half

10. Slice the avocados, use a spoon to remove the pit and the remainder of the fruit. Discard the pit and the skin

11. Place the eggs halves on a plate, top with avocado and then bacon

Scrambled Eggs with Cheese

Time: 10 Minutes | Serves 1
Macros: Calories: 327 | Fats: 31g | Carbs: 1g | Protein: 11g

Ingredients

♦ 2 large eggs
♦ ¼ cup water
♦ ¼ tbsp. butter
♦ Salt
♦ Pepper
♦ Shredded cheese (your choice)

Preparation

1. Break the eggs over a bowl and add some water to them

2. Scramble the eggs with a whisk, stirring forcefully until the yolks are broken and have been fully combined with the egg whites

3. Put a pan on the stove and allow it to heat up with some butter inside

4. Pour the eggs into the pan

5. Cook the eggs by moving them around in the pan with a spatula until they are fully cooked

6. Place the eggs on a plate. Add the salt, pepper, and cheese if you wish

Cauliflower Hash Browns

Time: 30 Minutes | Serves 2
Macros: Calories: 898 | Fats: 87g | Carbs: 9g | Protein: 17g

Ingredients

- 3 cups of cauliflower
- 4 tbsp butter
- 6 large eggs
- ½ cup of peppers, poblamo
- Salt
- Pepper
- 2/3 cup of mayonnaise
- 2 tbsp garlic salt

Preparation

1. Pulse the cauliflower in a food processor until it's completely broken down into bits

2. Pour the mayonnaise and the garlic salt into the cauliflower, mix thoroughly

3. Place a pan on the stove with the butter in it. Turn the heat on medium and wait until the butter is melting and sizzling

4. Saute the cauliflower in a pan, mixing thoroughly as it cooks

5. Remove the cauliflower from the pan and then place it in a bowl during the next steps

6. Cook the peppers the same way

7. Put the pepper in a bowl with the cauliflower

8. Place the eggs in the same pan and then cook them

9. Put the eggs on a plate and top with the cauliflower and peppers. Add some cheese and salt and pepper if you want

Tuna Salad And Hot Peppers

Time: 10 Minutes | Serves 1
Macros: Calories: 271 | Fats: 26g | Carbs: 1g | Protein: 8g

Ingredients

- 1 can tuna
- ½ cup chopped hot peppers (your choice)
- ¼ cup mayonnaise
- Pepper
- Salt

Preparation

1. Open the can of tuna and drain the water or oil from it

2. Put the tuna into a small bowl

3. Add the peppers to the bowl and stir until they are well mixed

4. Pour in the mayonnaise and stir

5. If you wish, add some salt and pepper

Scrambled Eggs Mexican-Style

Time: 20 Minutes | Serves 2
Macros: Calories: 229 | Fats: 18g | | Carbs: 2g | Protein: 14g

Ingredients

♦ 4 large eggs

♦ ¼ cup of water

♦ 3 jalapeno peppers, chopped

♦ 2 small tomatoes, chopped

♦ 1 onion that has been chopped thin

♦ 3 tbsp of butter

♦ Salt

♦ Pepper

♦ Shredded cheese

Preparation

1. Place a frying pan on the stove and turn the heat to medium. Put the butter in it. When the butter is sizzling and melted, move on to the next step

2. Place the peppers, onions, and tomatoes in the pan

3. Cook them until they are well browned

4. Take them out of the pan, but don't drain the butter and juices

5. Break the eggs into a bowl and then add the water

6. Scramble the eggs with a fork or a whisk, stirring forcefully until the yolks are broken and are thoroughly mixed with the egg whites

7. Pour the eggs into the pan

8. Use a spatula to move the eggs around in the pan until they are fully cooked

9. Add the other vegetables back into the pan

10. Put everything on a plate and put cheese on top

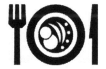

Keto Friendly Pancakes

Time: 20 Minutes | Serves 2
Macros: Calories: 425 | Fats: 39g | Carbs: 5g | Protein: 13g

Ingredients

♦ 3 large eggs
♦ 2small containersof cheese, cottage
♦ 3 tbsp psyllium husk
♦ 2 tbsp butter
♦ Salt
♦ Pepper

Preparation

1. Break the eggs into a bowl and then stir well until the yolks are broken and they are fully mixed with the egg whites

2. Add the syllium husks and the cottage cheese, allow the mixture to sit for 15 minutes

3. Place a frying pan on the stove over medium heat, melt the butter in it. When the butter is sizzling and melted, move on to the next step

4. Pour the eggs, cottage cheese, and psyllium husk to the pan and use your handsand form cakes

5. Flip them while cooking to keep them from sticking to the pan

6. Add some salt and pepper to the top of them

Recipes for Lunch

Egg Salad

Time: 30 Minutes | Serves 4
Macros Per Serving: Calories: 439 | Fats: 41g | Carbs: 3g | Protein: 12g

Ingredients

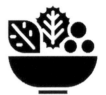

♦ 8 eggs

♦ 3 stalks of chopped celery

♦ 3 stalks of green onions

♦ 2 bell peppers

♦ 1 tbsp mustard

♦ ¾ cup of mayonnaise

♦ Salt and pepper

Preparation

1. Place the eggs (shells and all) in a cooking pot

2. Add water to the pot until all of the eggs are covered and there is one inch of clearance (note: the eggs will float)

3. Place the pan on the stove and turn the heat onto high

4. Once the water boils, set a cooking timer for ten minutes

5. Slice the eggs before mashing them

6. Stir in the celery, green onion, and green bell pepper.

7. Stir in the mayonnaise and mustard.

8. Add salt and pepper if you wish

Zucchini and Sausage Boats

Time: 50 Minutes | Serves 4
Macros: Calories: 536 | Fats: 45.35g | Carbs: 5.82g | Protein: 24.38g

Ingredients

♦ 1 cup of ground sausage

♦ 3 zucchini

♦ 1 package of the shredded cheese of your choice (cheddar works well)

♦ ¼ of a medium sized onion

♦ 2 tbsp garlic, minced

♦ 2 tsp paprika

♦ ½ tbsp of red pepper flakes

♦ 2 tsp oregano1 cup of chicken stock or broth

♦ Salt and pepper

Preparation

1. Preheat the oven to 350 degrees F/176 degrees C

2. Slice the zucchini in half and remove the inside sections in order to create zucchini shells

3. Place the removed part of the zucchini, as well as the other Ingredients (minus the sausage), to a pan and cook them until they are browned

4. Add the sausage to the same pan, and then cook it until it is done

5. Put the zucchini shells in a baking pan

6. Put the sausage mixture inside of them

7. Sprinkle cheese on top

8. Put the chicken broth in the center of the pan around the zucchini

9. Place it in the oven for around 30 minutes

Meatless Keto Club Salad

Time: 10 Minutes | Serves 1
Macros: Calories: 329.67 | Fats: 26.32g | Carbs: 4.83g | Protein: 16.82g

Ingredients

- 3 tbsp of sour cream
- 3 tbsp of mayonnaise
- 1 tsp milk
- 1/4 tsp garlic salt
- ½ tsp onion powder
- 2 tsp dried basil
- 2 tsp parsley
- 3 hard boiled eggs, sliced
- 4 ounces cheddar cheese, cubed
- 3 cups of shredded lettuce
- ½ cup of tomatoes
- 1 cup cucumber
- 2tsp of mustard

Preparation

1. Mix the Ingredients (minus the eggs) in a small container

2. Place the eggs (shells and all) in a cooking pot

3. Add water to the pot until all of the eggs are covered and there is one inch of clearance (note: the eggs will float)

4. Place the pan on the stove and turn the heat onto high

5. Once the water boils, set a cooking timer for ten minutes

6. Slice and then mash the eggs.

7. Arrange the eggs, lettuce, tomatoes, cucumber, and Dijon mustard on a plate or in a bowl

8. Pour the dressing over the salad

9. Top with cheese

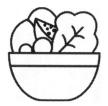

Eggplant and Cheese Keto "Bread"

Time: 35 Minutes | Serves 3
Macros: Calories: 194 | Fats: 14.23g | Carbs: 5.73g | Protein: 8g

Ingredients

♦ 2 baby eggplants, cubed

♦ 1 package of the shredded cheese of your choice (mozzarella works well)

♦ 2 tsp garlic powder

♦ ¼ tsp basil

♦ 3 tbsp butter

Preparation

1. Set the oven to 375 degrees F/190 degrees C

2. Mix the garlic powder and basil in with the butter

3. Divide the cubed eggplant into three equal servings, place them at the bottom of three sections of a muffin pan

4. Coat the eggplant with the cheese

5. Spoon the butter and seasonings over the cheese and the eggplant

6. Put in the oven for 15 to 20 minutes

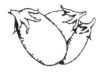

Mushroom and Cauliflower Grits

Time: 20 Minutes | Serves 4
Macros: Calories: 455 | Fats: 36.5g | Carbs: 11.28g | Protein: 15.28g

Ingredients

♦ 1 cupmushrooms
♦ 5 cloves of minced garlic
♦ 2 tbsp rosemary
♦ ¼ cup of walnuts that have been chopped
♦ 2 tbsp paprika
♦ 3 tsp of olive oil
♦ 588 g cauliflower, chopped
♦ ½ cup water
♦ 2 cups of creamer
♦ 1 package of the shredded cheese of your choice
♦ 3 tbsp butter
♦ Salt

Preparation

1. Set the oven on 400 degrees F/ or 204 degrees C

2. Lay the mushrooms and walnuts on a baking sheet, sprinkle with garlic, paprika, rosemary, salt, and olive oil

3. Place in the oven for ten to fifteen minutes

4. Place the cauliflower in a food processor or blender. Break into small pieces

5. Steam the cauliflower over water until it is tender and ready to eat

6. Pour the cauliflower into a pan and then add in the creamer. Cook on low

7. Add cheese and other Ingredients (minus the mushrooms) into the pan and stir them together

8. Pour the cauliflower "grits" into a bowl and top with mushrooms

Keto Caprese Salad

Time: 40 Minutes | Serves 1
Macros: Calories: 190.75 | Fats: 63.49g | Carbs: 4.58g | Protein: 7.79g

Ingredients

- 5 cloves of minced garlic or garlic salt
- 4 cups of tomatoes that have been chopped
- 3 tbsp avocado oil
- 4 cups baby spinach
- 10 pieces mozzarella balls
- 1 tbsp pesto
- 1 tbsp brine, mozzarella brine
- ¼ cup basil

Preparation

1. Set the oven to 400 degrees/204 degrees C
2. Lay garlic and tomatoes on a lined baking sheet and then place the avocado oil on top of them
3. Bake for 30 minutes
4. Mix the mozzarella brine with the pesto to make a dressing
5. Place the spinach and roasted garlic and tomatoes in a bowl
6. Top with mozzarella cheese (break it into chunks first), and then the vegetable mixture
7. Put the dressing on it

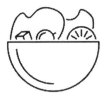

Keto Taco Salad

Time:30Minutes | Serves 4
Macros: Calories: 250 | Fats: 25g | Carbs: 2.35g | Protein: 15g

Ingredients

- 1 cup of ground beef
- 1 cup of water
- Chopped lettuce
- Chopped tomatoes
- 2 avocadoes
- 2 tbsp taco seasoning
- Shredded cheese of your choice

Preparation

1. Put the pan on the stove over medium heat. When the pan has heated and is slightly smoking, place the beef in it

2. Brown the meat in the pan, stirring as needed, when it's cooked, drain the grease and move on to the next step

3. Add water to the meat and then include the taco seasoning, stirring thoroughly. Then, let the meat and seasoning mixture to cook until it is heated all of the way through

4. Put the ground beef on a plate. Top it with lettuce that has been shredded, tomatoes, avocado, and cheese. Wait a few minutes for the cheese to melt before serving

5. If you'd like, add some pepper and salt

Avocado and Chicken Salad

Time:20Minutes | Serves 1
Macros: Calories: 550 | Fats: 38g | Carbs: 10g | Protein: 40g

Ingredients

- 1 cup chicken, already cooked and shredded
- ½ medium sized cucumber
- 1 avocado
- 4 small tomatoes (cherry tomatoes work well)
- 2 small onions
- 3 tsp lime or lemon juice or zest
- 3 tbsp olive oil
- Pepper
- Salt

Preparation

1. Prepare the vegetables by chopping them into small pieces

2. Slice the avocado. Discard the skin and the pit, as you won't need them

3. Put the lemon or lime juice or zest into a bowl with the olive oil and mix them together

4. Place the shredded chicken on a platewithout cooking it further, as it should be cold. Then, add the veggies on top of it. (Note: this is a useful method of using up leftovers from the night before)

5. Put the olive oil and juice mixture onto the chicken and veggies and then mix them together

6. Add salt and pepper to taste

Egg Salad with Avocado

Time:20Minutes | Serves 4
Macros: Calories: 250 | Fats: 52.5g | Carbs: 2.53g | Protein: 8.65g

Ingredients

- ◆ 6 large eggs
- ◆ 3 tbsp of lemon or lime juice
- ◆ 3 avocados
- ◆ 1 small red onion
- ◆ 3 tsp dill
- ◆ Salt
- ◆ Pepper

Preparation

1. Place the eggs (shells and all) in a cooking pot

2. Add water to the pot until all of the eggs are covered and there is one inch of clearance (note: the eggs will float)

3. Place the pan on the stove and turn the heat onto high

4. Once the water boils, set a cooking timer for ten minutes

5. Allow the eggs to cool before peeling them

6. 6)Take the pit and the skin off of the avocadoes and mash them

7. Chop the red onion into small pieces

8. Slice the eggs into chunks

9. Mix the mashed avocado, red onion, eggs, and seasonings together

10. Serve

Chili

Time:45Minutes | Serves 6
Macros: Calories: 306 | Fats: 18g | Carbs: 13g | Protein: 23g

Ingredients

♦ 1 package of your choice of ground beef

♦ 1 can diced chilis and tomatoes

♦ Premade chili seasoning

♦ 1 jar of tomato sauce

♦ 2 medium sized onions, diced

♦ Salt

♦ Pepper

Preparation

1. Put a deep pan on the stove over medium heat. When it's slightly smoking, put the ground beef, onion, and diced tomatoes and chilis in it (Note: chili usually has beans in it, but since beans are high in carbs, this version does not include them)

2. Add salt and pepper while the meat is still cooking. When the beef is browned it is done. Continue to stir as needed until this state has been reached

3. Make sure to drain the grease from the meat before moving on to the next step

4. Place the seasonings and tomato sauce into the pan

5. Let the chili boil and then turn it down low so that it can simmer.

6. Allow to simmer until everything is cooked through

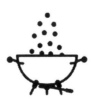

Beef Stew

Time: 40 Minutes | Serves 1
Macros: | Calories: 288 | Fats: 20g | Carbs: 8g | Protein: 20g

Ingredients

- 3 cups of beef, can be roast, stir fry meat, stew meat, or whatever you choose
- 1.5 containers of beef stock
- 2 heads of celery
- 2 medium sized onions
- 5 cloves of minced garlic
- 3 small carrots
- 3 small turnips
- 2 tbsp parsley
- 1 tbsp basil
- Salt
- Pepper

Preparation

1. Prepare the meat by cutting it into small chunks if necessary

2. Chop all of the vegetables in small pieces

3. Place the meat in a stew pot. Add in the garlic and onions, as well as the salt and pepper

4. Sauté the beef. Once it is full cooked, move on to the next step

5. Pour in the beef stock and all of the vegetables, and then stir well (Note: since quite a few of the veggies listed here are high-carb root vegetables, only use a small number of them)

6. Allow the stew to boil and then turn it down to low so that it can simmer for several hours. Once the vegetables are soft, it's ready

7. Salt and pepper to taste

Lettuce Wrapped Cheeseburgers

Time:30Minutes | Serves 4
Macros: Calories: 353 | Fats: 56.5g | Carbs: 2.5g | Protein: 30.9g

Ingredients

♦ 2 cups of the ground beef of your choice

♦ 1 egg that has been scrambled

♦ 1/2 small onion

♦ Salt

♦ 3 cloves garlic

♦ Pepper

♦ Iceberg lettuce

♦ Sliced cheese of your choice

Preparation

1. Chop the garlic and the onion until they are in very small pieces

2. Put the ground beef in a bowl and add the remaining Ingredients, except for the lettuce and the cheese. Mix well

3. Arrange the meat so that it's in small balls that can be mashed flat

4. Place a pan on the stove over medium heat. Once it heats up, place the burger patties on it

5. Flip the meat patties are they cook in order to ensure that they are fried all of the way through, pressing down on occasion to keep them together

6. Prepare the lettuce by washing it and gently peeling off several large leaves

7. Top the patty with cheese and wrap in lettuce. You can also serve with mayonnaise

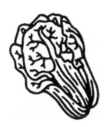

Healthy Green Smoothie

Time:10Minutes | Serves 1
Macros: Calories: 340 | Fats: 24.7g | Carbs: 25.1g | Protein: 5.6g

Ingredients

♦ 2 cups spinach

♦ 1 avocado

♦ ¾ cup of milk (coconut milk works well)

♦ ½ cup water

♦ 2 tsp of extract, vanilla

♦ 2 tbsp matcha powder

♦ 1 tbsp sweetener

♦ 6 ice cubes

♦ 1 cup water

Preparation

1. Prepare the spinach by washing it and breaking it into very small pieces

2. Slice the avocado, removing the pit and skin

3. Put the remaining Ingredients into a blender

4. Turn the blender on and allow it to run until the contents are smooth

5. Serve

Keto-Friendly Chicken Sandwich

Time: 40 Minutes | Serves 4
Macros: Calories: 405 | Fats: 31g | Carbs: 6.72g | Protein: 24.8g

Ingredients

- 1 package cream cheese
- 4 large eggs
- 1/3 tbsp. cream of tartar
- 1 tbsp garlic salt
- 4 tbsp mayonnaise
- 2 tbsp sriracha sauce1 chunked cooked, cold chicken breast
- 4 pieces cooked bacon
- Sliced cheese of your choice
- 2 small sliced tomatoes

Preparation

1. Preheat oven to 300 degrees F/148 degrees C

2. Place the eggs into a bowl, add the salt, cream of tartar, garlic powder, and cream cheese, then mix thoroughlyPut wax paper on a baking sheet

3. Pour the eggs and the related mixture onto the wax paper, forming small, even circles of batter

4. Bake for 30 minutes

5. Combine the sauces (sriracha and mayonnaise) in a bowl and stir until thoroughly combined

6. Put the chicken on the "bread" that has just emerged from the oven, top with bacon, tomatoes, and the mixed sauce

Crock Pot Pizza

Time:4 Hours | Serves 8
Macros: Calories: 400 | Fats: 56.2g | Carbs: 2.36g | Protein: 25.4g

Ingredients

- 1 package ground beef
- 2 tbsp garlic powder
- 1 onion
- Salt
- Pepper
- 1 can pizza or tomato sauce
- 1 package shredded cheese of your choice (mozzarella works well)
- Pepperoni
- Mushrooms
- Any other pizza toppings that you like

Preparation

1. Prepare the onion by chopping it into small pieces

2. Place a pan on the stove over medium heat, when it's fully heated and smoking slightly, put the ground beef in it

3. Place the additional Ingredients (not the toppings) in with the ground beef and mix thoroughly

4. Cook the ground beef, stirring as needed, until full cooked

5. Wash and slice the mushrooms

6. Remove the grease from the ground beef

7. Put the meat into the crock pot

8. Top with pepperoni, mushrooms, cheese, sauce, and any of the other toppings

9. If you'd like, season with pepper and salt

10. Set the crock pot on low, when the cheese melts and begins to bubble, it's done

Recipes for Dinner

Skillet Enchilada Chicken

Time: 40 Minutes | Serves 4
Macros: Calories: 273.75 | Fats: 13.98g | Carbs: 2.81g | Protein: 31.93g

Ingredients

♦ 1 lb chicken breasts, sliced in half

♦ ½ cup of flour, almond

♦ 2 tbsp butter

♦ 3 eggs

♦ ½ cup red enchilada sauce

♦ ¼ cup of the shredded cheese of your choice

♦ 1/3 cup of diced onion

♦ Salt and pepper

♦ Cilantro

Preparations

1. Crack the eggs into a bowl and then mix them until they are slightly scrambled

2. Put each piece of chicken individually into a bowl, then press into almond flour

3. Preheat the oven to 400 degrees F/204 degrees C

4. Place a pan on thestove top, turn it on, and melt the butter into it

5. Cook the chicken in the pan for about seven minutes per side

6. Transfer the chicken into a baking dish that is over safe

7. Pour the sauce on the chicken and the follow with the onion and cheese

8. Sprinkle the cilantro and salt and pepper on top, if desired

9. Bake in the oven for around 30 minutes

Zucchini with Walnut Pesto

Time: 20 Minutes | Serves 2
Macros: Calories: 325.5 | Fats: 26.08g | Carbs: 11.46g | Protein: 10.65g

Ingredients

- 3 medium zucchini, sliced into ribbons
- ½ teaspoon salt
- ½ large avocado
- 1 cup basil1 cup walnuts
- 3 cloves of garlic
- ½ large lemon
- 2 tbsp of olive oil
- Pepper
- Salt
- 1/3 cup of the cheese of your choice (preferably parmesan)

Preparation

1. Toss the zucchini ribbons into a bowl with the salt and allow it to sit for around ten minutes

2. While the zucchini sits, place the avocado, basil, walnuts, garlic, cheese and lemon in a blender and then turn it on to form the pesto.

3. Place a frying pan on the stove and pour in the olive oil, once it's ready (it will sizzle), add zucchini, and cook it until it's nice and tender. Remove from heat

4. Put the zucchini into a bowl and then add the pesto. Stir in order to coat the zucchini with the pesto

5. Add salt and pepper to taste before serving

Cauliflower Salad

Time: 10 Minutes | Serves 10
Macros: Calories: 211.12 | Fats: 19.6g | Carbs: 2.82g | Protein: 4.92g

Ingredients

- 1 medium head cauliflower, chopped
- 4 hard boiled eggs, chopped
- 1 cup mayonnaise
- ⅓ cup bacon bits
- 2 tbsp apple cider vinegar
- ¼ cup onions, chopped
- 1 tsp garlic, minced
- ¾ cup of chopped green onions
- 1 tsp sugar substitute

Preparation

1. Combine the eggs, mayonnaise, bacon bits, apple cider vinegar, onions, garlic, sugar substitute, and green onions in a bowl. Stir until everything in the bowl is fully combined

2. Slowly stir in the cauliflower until everything is blended together

3. Serve cold

Keto Spinach and Watercress Salad

Time: 10 Minutes | Serves 4
Macros: Calories: 203.75 | Fats: 18.59g | Carbs: 1.85g | Protein: 5.32g

Ingredients

♦ 2cups of watercress that have been cleaned, prepared, and ready to use

♦ 3 cups baby spinach, cleaned and stemmed

♦ 1 avocado that has been sliced

♦ ½ cup of the shredded cheese of your choice

♦ ¼ cup avocado oil

♦ Salt

♦ Pepper

♦ Lemon or lime juice

Preparation

1. Mix the oil, the lemon or lime juice, and the salt and pepper (if you wish to use them) in a bowl to make the dressing

2. Put the spinach and watercress into a small bowl

3. Put the avocado on top of them

4. Drizzle on the dressing

5. Sprinkle your shredded cheese on top

Zucchini Nests

Time: 40 Minutes | Serves 6
Macros: Calories: 130.83 | Fats: 9.88g | Carbs: 4.27g | Protein: 5.97g

Ingredients

♦ 4 small zucchinis, cut into spiral patterns

♦ ¼ cup cheddar cheese, shredded

♦ 1/3 cup onion, chopped into small pieces

♦ 6 pieces of cooked bacon

♦ 2 tsp garlic powder

♦ 15 tbsp of sour cream

♦ Salt and pepper

Preparation

1. Preheat the oven to 350 degrees F/176 degrees C

2. Lay the spiral shaped zucchini pieces on a greased cookie or baking sheet so that they resemble bird's nests or spiral shapes

3. Place some salt, pepper, and garlic powder on top of them

4. Top with the onion, bacon, and cheese

5. Bake for 30 minutes

6. Top with sour cream if you desire

Keto Cheeseburger and Bacon Casserole

Time: 60 Minutes | Serves 12
Macros Per Serving: Calories: 548 | Fats: 36.6g | Carbs: 4.4g | Protein: 48.5g

Ingredients

- 2 packages of ground beef
- 1 package of bacon that has been cooked and chopped
- 8 eggs, raw and shelled
- 3 cloves of minced garlic
- 1/3 tsp of garlic salt
- 1 can of tomato paste
- 1 cup of whipping cream
- 1 package of the shredded cheese of your choice
- Salt and pepper

Preparation

1. Preheat the oven to 350 degrees F/176 degrees C

2. Place the ground meat in a pan along with the garlic, and salt and pepper. Brown the meat

3. After draining off any of the extra grease, put the cooked ground beef into a casserole dish that has been properly greased

4. Pour the eggs, heavy cream, tomato paste, and around half of the cheese into a large bowl. Mix well.

5. Place the egg mixture on top of the meat mixture and stir

6. Put the remainder of the cheese on top of this mixture

7. Bake for 30 minutes.

Garlic Seasoned Scallops

Time: 30 Minutes | Serves 3
Macros Per Serving: Calories: 418 | Fats: 8g | Carbs: 4g | Protein: 49g

Ingredients

- 1 pound scallops, cleaned
- 1 tbsp lemon juice
- 2 cloves minced garlic
- 2 tbsp parsley
- 1 tsp of butter
- 2 tbsp extra virgin olive oil
- 2 tbsp red pepper flakes
- 1 tsp paprika
- Pepper
- Salt

Preparation

1. Put the olive oil in a frying pan on the stove. Heat it very slowly in order to avoid harming the oil. Once it begins to heat up, increase the heat on the burner. When it starts to sizzle, then it is ready.

2. Place the lemon juice, parsley, butter, red pepper flakes, and other seasonings into a bowl. Add salt and pepper to taste. Add in the scallops, treating them very gently. Stir to coat the scallops thoroughly in the seasoning

3. Place the scallops in the frying pan. Turn them every few minutes. They may only need to cook for four to five minutes

4. Cook the scallops until they are golden brown

Salmon With Miso

Time: 55 Minutes | Serves 4
Macros: Calories: 215.25 | Fats: 9.23g | Carbs: .78g | Protein: 28.38g

Ingredients

♦ 5 salmon fillets (make sure that they have the skin still attached at the bottom)

♦ Kosher salt3 tbsp sake

♦ 4 tbsp of white wine (your choice of wine)

♦ 4 tbsp miso

Preparation

1. If the salmon is not already filleted, carefully cut it into portions using a good knife. Be very careful as salmon is a tender fish and you don't want to harm it.

2. Sprinkle the salt onto the top of the salmon. Place it aside and let it sit for around 20 minutes.

3. Preheat the oven to 400 degrees F/204 degrees C

4. Mix the remaining Ingredients (the salt, sake, miso, and white wine) in a small mixing bowl until well combined

5. Place a thin coat of the mixture onto the salmon, drizzling it in a controlled fashion, and then gently press is on with your fingertips

6. Put the salmon fillets on a baking sheet

7. Put the salmon in the oven and bake it for around 30 minutes, or until it is flaky. Do not overbake

8. Serve with your favorite Keto-friendly side dish

Lemon Fish Fillets

Time: 20 Minutes | Serves 2
Macros: Calories: 406 | Fats: 30.33g | Carbs: 3.55g | Protein: 29.07g

Ingredients

- 2 fillets of the fishof your choice
- 5 tbsp of butter
- 2 tbsp of lime or lemon zest or juice
- 1/3 cup of flour, almond
- 2 tsp dill
- 1 tsp chives
- 1 tbsp garlic salt
- 1 tbsp onion power
- Pepper
- Salt

Preparation

1. Place all of the Ingredients except for the fish (some of the butter, lime or lemon zest or juice, flour, chives, garlic salt, onion powder, and dill) into a bowl and mix until combined

2. Put the remaining butter into a microwave safe bowl and melt

3. Put each piece of fish into the butter, submerging it entirely. Then place it into the batter bowl. Shake it slightly to ensure that the batter is not going to come off

4. Sprinkle any of the excess batter on top of the fish once you have laid them in the pan

5. Put some of the lime or lemon zest or juice in the bottom of a pan, along with an extra pat of butter

6. Sauté the fish thoroughly, flipping it as needed, until it is fully cooked

Keto Tuna Casserole

Time: 55 Minutes | Serves 6
Macros: Calories: 248.5 | Fats: 21.21g | Carbs: 3.07g | Protein: 10.28g

Ingredients

- ◆ 2 tbsp of butter
- ◆ ½ cup of carrots
- ◆ 2/3 cup of mushrooms
- ◆ 2/3 cup of green onions
- ◆ 1.5 cups of cream, heavy whipping
- ◆ ¼ tsp xanthan gum
- ◆ 226g zucchini noodles
- ◆ 1 cup of cheese of your choice, shredded
- ◆ 2 cans of tuna
- ◆ Salt and pepper

Preparation

1. Put the butter in a pan and place it on medium heat
2. Add in the Ingredients except for the tuna, whipping cream, and noodles and then cook them until they are tender
3. Add in the whipping cream, and then cook slowly until the mixture has thickened
4. Set the oven on 350 degrees F/176 degrees C
5. Spread the zucchini noodles out in a greased casserole dish
6. Add the remaining mixture on top of the noodles
7. Add the tuna, as well as the salt and pepper, stirring until combined

8. Top with cheddar cheese

9. Bake for 35 minutes

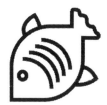

Stuffed Beef Rolls

Time: 40 Minutes | Serves 2
Macros: Calories: 423.5 | Fats: 31.79g | Carbs: 5.63g | Protein: 25.39g

Ingredients

- 1 flank steak that has been sliced thin
- 25 grams prosciutto
- 1 package of cream cheese
- 1 package of mozzarella cheese, shredded
- 2 tbsp of grated parmesan cheese
- 25 grams the shredded cheese of your choice
- 3 tbsp butter
- 100 grams mushrooms, chopped
- 3 tsp garlic, minced
- 1/3 cup of onion, chopped
- Pepper
- Salt

Preparations

1. Preheat oven to 375 degrees F/190 degrees C

2. Place the onion, mushrooms, and roughly half of the butter in a pan

3. Sauté until tender

4. Take the pan off of the stove and then stir in the cream cheese, mixing well

5. Add in the remaining cheeses and allow to melt thoroughly, stirring ocassionally

6. Lay the meat flat on a cutting board in layers with the prosciutto on the bottom and the flank steak on top

7. Place the mushroom mixture with the cheese on top of the flattened meat

8. Place some of the filling on each piece of meat and then roll them to form a tube

9. Melt the other section of butter in a pan

10. Saute the meat until the cheese has melted and the meat is fully cooked. This will take around 15 to 20 minutes

Shrimp Alfredo

Time: 30 Minutes | Serves 4
Macros: Calories: 297.83 | Fats: 17.55g | Carbs: 6.51g | Protein: 22.93g

Ingredients

- 1 tbsp butter, salted
- 1 package of shrimp that has been cleaned and shelled
- 1 package of cream cheese cut into cubes
- ½ cup whole milk
- 1 tbsp garlic powder
- 1 tsp basil
- 1 tsp salt
- ½ cup Parmesan cheese, shredded
- 5 whole sun dried tomatoes, sliced
- ¼ cup baby kale
- zucchini noodles for serving

Preparations

1. Melt butter in a skillet. Once it starts to sizzle, add the shrimp

2. Sprinkle seasoning salt onto the shrimp. Flip them over and then season again. They only need to cook for a few moments, particularly if you use precooked shrimp. Once they are tender, move on to the next step.

3. Add cream cheese and milk, stir until melted and creamy

4. Add in garlic powder, basil, salt and parmesan cheese, stir until melted

5. Stir in the tomatoes and kale

6. Serve with zucchini noodles

Taco Soup

Time: 5 Hours | Serves 8
Macros: Calories: 398 | Fats: 29g | Carbs: 6.9g | Protein: 28.5g

Ingredients

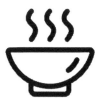

- 1 package ground beef
- ½ tsp red pepper flakes
- 2 tbsp of chili powder
- 2 tsp cumin
- 3 tsp red pepper flakes
- ½ tsp oregano
- Salt
- Pepper
- 2 packages of cream cheese
- 2 cans diced tomatoes
- 1 can of green chilis that have been diced
- 2 containers beef broth
- ½ cup heavy whipping cream

Preparations

1. Brown the ground beef on the stovetop in a pan, stirring until every piece of it is cooked thoroughly. Drain the excess grease (depending on the fat content of the meat used, you may not need to do this) and then place the beef into a crockpot

2. Add in the additional Ingredients, starting with the seasonings. Finish by stirring the whipping cream and the beef broth into the slow cooker

3. Place the slow cooker's lid on and then set it on high for four hours

4. Serve and enjoy

Oven Baked Pork Chops with Salad

Time: 45 Minutes | Serves 2
Macros: Calories: 325 | Fats: 15.25g | Carbs: 5.67g | Protein: 52.3g

Ingredients

- 2 boneless pork chops
- 1 tsp pepper
- 1 tsp salt
- 1 tbsp garlic salt
- 1 tbsp dried parsley
- 1 tbsp dried basil
- 2 cups of lettuce
- 2 cups of spinach
- Cherry tomatoes
- Olive oil as necessary

Preparations

1. Place the pork chops a baking pan that is nonstick

2. Sprinkle them on all sides with the seasonings – garlic salt, parsley, basil, salt, and pepper, in that order

3. Bake at 350 degrees F/176 degrees C until fully cooked and interior has reach a temperature of 165 degrees F/73 degrees C

4. Wash both the spinach and the lettuce. Shred them into tiny pieces and then mix with your hands stopping only when they are well combined. Prepare the cherry tomatoes by removing the stem and slicing them in half. Put the tomatoes on top of the spinach and lettuce

5. Pour a little of the olive oil on top of the salad that you have just made

6. Place the pork chops on a plate with the salad next to them

Keto Meatloaf

Time:85 Minutes | Serves 6
Macros: Calories: 344 | Fats: 29g | Carbs: 4g | Protein: 33g

Ingredients

- 2 package of beef, ground
- 3 eggs
- 4 garlic cloves
- 2/3 cup yeast
- 1 tsp pepper
- 3 tbsp avocado oil
- 1/3 cup of fresh or dried parsley
- 1 tbsp lemon or lime zest
- ¼ cup of oregano (fresh or dried)

Preparations

1. Crack the eggs into a blender. Add in the avocado oil, all of the herbs (minus the salt and pepper), and the garlic. Blend until everything is well mixed and a creamy batter is formed

2. Put the ground beef in a bowl and sprinkle with the salt and pepper. Use your hands to mix everything together

3. Pour the egg mixture into the bowl with the ground beef mixture. Combine them thoroughly

4. Preheat the oven to 400 degrees F/204 degrees C

5. Move the entire mixture into a nonstick baking loaf pan. Make sure that the loaf is even on all sides

6. Bake for one hour or until fully cooked

7. Serve with a green salad or the side dish of your choice

Recipes for Snacks and Desserts

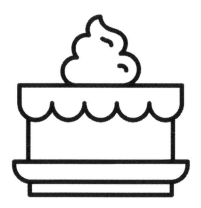

Macadamia Nut Fat Bombs

Time: 10 Minutes | Serves 6
Macros Per Serving: Calories: 99 | Fats: 16.9g | Carbs: 1.9g | Protein: 0.8g

Ingredients

♦ 10 nuts, preferably macadamia, although you can substitute others

♦ 3 tbsp cocoa powder, unsweetened

♦ 2 tsp extract, vanilla

♦ 3 tbsp erythriol

♦ 1/3 cup room temperature unrefined coconut oil

♦ Salt

Preparation

1. Combine vanilla extract, cocoa powder, erythritol, and oil of coconut into a bowl. Mix well until the batter is very smooth

2. Arrange wax paper on the sides and bottom of a small freezable container. Wax paper will work as well. Press down hard to ensure that the paper stays in place

3. Pour the cocoa powder mixture into the freezable container

4. Place the macadamia nuts on the top part of mixture while it isthe lined container, followed by a light sprinkling of salt

5. Place the mixture in the freezer for several minutes or until semi-hard, then slice into 6 squares. These can be kept in the freezer until you are ready for them. Make sure to slice them before they are fully frozen

Keto Zucchini Bread

Time: 70 Minutes | Serves 16
Macros: Calories: 200.13 | Fats: 18.83g | Carbs: 2.6g | Protein: 5.59g

Ingredients

♦ 3 eggs
♦ ¼ cup of olive oil, extra virgin
♦ 2 tsp of vanilla extract
♦ 3 cups of flour, almond
♦ 2 cups of erythritol
♦ 1/3 tsp of salt
♦ 2 tbsp baking powder
♦ 1/3 tsp of nutmeg
♦ 2 tsp cinnamon, ground
♦ 1/3 tsp ginger, ground
♦ 2 cup zucchini, grated
♦ ½ cup walnuts, chopped

Preparation

1. Preheat the oven to 350 degrees F/176 degrees C

2. Pour eggs, oil, and vanilla extract into a bowl, stir until everything is well mixed

3. Using a separate bowl, place the almond flour, erythritol, salt, baking powder, nutmeg, ginger, and ground cinnamon until combined

4. Wrap the zucchini slices in several towels or pieces of cheesecloth. Squeeze gently until they are dry

5. Add zucchini to the eggs mixture and then stir everything well until the zucchini pieces are coated

6. Pour the combined Ingredients into one single bowl, stir until well mixed

7. Using a greased baking pan, add the batter in an even layer

8. Sprinkle the walnuts on the cake before it goes into the oven

9. Bake for 60 minutes

Matcha Cheesecake

Time: 70 Minutes | Serves 6
Macros: Calories: 350.33 | Fats: 33.24g | Carbs: 5.81g | Protein: 8.46g

Ingredients

- 1 package of cream cheese
- 1/3 cup of non-sugar swcetener
- 3 tbsp flour, coconut
- ½ tsp extract, vanilla
- 3 tbsp cream, heavy whipping
- 2 tsp matcha powder
- 2 eggs
- ¼ cup of sour cream
- 2 tbsp non-sugar sweetener

Preparation

1. Set the oven to 300 degrees F/148 degrees C

2. Put the cream cheese, sugar substitute, coconut flour, vanilla extract, whipping cream, and matcha in a bowl and then stir very well

3. Crack the eggs one at a time into the bowl, stirring as you add them

4. Pour the mixture into a greased, round baking pan

5. Bake for 50 minutes

6. Combined the sugar substitute and the sour cream together

7. Place the sour cream mixture on top of the cake after it has fully cooled

8. Place the cake in the refrigerator for three hours before serving

Flourless Brownies

Time: 40 Minutes | Serves 16
Macros: Calories: 86.94 | Fats: 8.05g | Carbs: 2.9g | Protein: 2.18g

Ingredients

♦ 1 cup of low-carb milk chocolate

♦ 4 tbsp of butter

♦ 4 large eggs

♦ ½ cup sugar substitute

♦ ¼ cup mascarpone cheese

♦ 1/3 cup of cocoa powder, unsweetened

♦ ½ tsp salt

Preparation

1. Preheat oven to 375 degrees F/190 degrees C

2. Place the chocolate in a microwavable bowl, melt it in the microwave 30 seconds at a time

3. Add the butter to the chocolate, microwave for 20 seconds until everything is completely melted

4. Place the sugar substitute and eggs in a bowl and then mix until thoroughly combined

5. Add the mascarpone cheese into the bowl with the sugar and eggs, mix thoroughly

6. Mix in the cocoa powder, then the add the remaining batter and stir well

7. Add the batter to a baking pan that has been well greased

8. Bake for 45 minutes

Coconut Chip Cookies

Time: 30 Minutes | Serves 16
Macros: Calories: 192.38 | Fats: 17.44g | Carbs: 2.17g | Protein: 4.67g

Ingredients

- 2 cups of flour, almond
- ½ cup cacao nibs¼ cup coconut flakes, unsweetened
- 1/3 cup of non-sugar sweetener or erythritol
- ¼ cup of nut butter (almond works best)
- 1/3 cup of butter, melted
- 3 eggs
- Liquid stevia or another type of non-sugar sweetener
- 1/3 tsp salt

Preparation

1. Preheat the oven to 350 degrees F/176 degrees C

2. Mix the almond butter, butter, eggs and liquid stevia in a bowl

3. Place the almond flour, cacao nibs, salt, erythritol, and coconut flakesin a different bowl and mix well

4. Combine the liquid Ingredients with the solid ones, mixing well

5. Portion the cookies out onto a lined sheet, flatten them out

6. Back for 20 minutes

Peanut Butter and Coconut Balls

Time: 70 Minutes | Serves 15
Macros: Calories: 35.13 | Fats: 3.19g | Carbs: .92g | Protein: .98g

Ingredients

- 3 tbsp peanut butter
- 3 tsp unsweetened cocoa powder
- 2 ½ tsp erythritol
- 2 tsp almond flour
- ½ cup unsweetened shredded coconut

Preparation

1. Combine the peanut butter, cocoa powder, erythritol, and almond flour in a bowl

2. Freeze for one hour in bowl

3. Scoop out 1/15 of the batter, roll in coconut, then shape into a ball

4. Refrigerate until eaten

Sugarless Cheesecake

Time: 8Hours | Serves 10
Macros: Calories: 100.15 | Fats: 5.29g | Carbs: .57g | Protein: .32g

Ingredients

- 1/2 cup of coconut, shredded
- ¼ cup of flour, coconut
- 1/3 cup flour, almond
- 3 blocks cream cheese
- 3 tsp almond extract
- 1 cup butter
- 2/3 cup sour cream
- 4 tsp vanilla extract
- 2 tbsp stevia
- 3 eggs

Preparation

1. Make the crust by placing the dry Ingredients (coconut, flours, almond extract, and butter) into a bowl and mixing them until they are well combined

2. Preheat the oven to 300 degrees F/148 degrees C

3. Grease the bottom of a small cake pan

4. Press the crust into the cake pan making sure to coat the bottom

5. Put the pan into the refrigerator

6. Place the rest of the ingredient into a bowl. This will be the vanilla extract, cream cheese, stevia, eggs, and other remaining Ingredients. Mix until smooth, then pour it over the crust

7. Bake the cake for one hour until the center jiggles slightly

8. Allow to cool completely before placing the cheesecake in the refrigerator overnight

9. Slice before serving

Coconut Ice Cream

Time: 5Hours | Serves 10
Macros: Calories: 130.25 | Fats: 6.35g | Carbs: .65g | Protein: .25g

Ingredients

- 3 cups of heavy cream for whipping
- 1 cup keto-friendly confectioner sugar
- 2 cans coconut milk
- 1/8 tsp salt
- 1.5 tsp vanilla extract

Preparation

1. Place the coconut milk in the refrigerator overnight to ensure that it is cooled and ready to use

2. The next day, open the cans. Separate the top layer of the coconut cream from the milk and put it into a bowl. You should be able to do this with a spoon

3. Pour the whipping cream, the salt, and the vanilla extract in a separate bowl. Beat with a mixer until creamy

4. Beat the coconut cream in its own bowl until creamy

5. Combine the coconut cream with the whipping cream mixture and mix well, but not to the point of liquefying either of them

6. Scoop the combined mixture into a pan.

7. Put the pan with the Ingredients intoa freezer. Freeze for five hours

Raspberry and Vanilla Keto Smoothie

Time:10 Minutes | Serves1
Macros: Calories: 552 | Fats: 55g | Carbs: 5.8g | Protein: 7.8g

Ingredients

- ½ cup raspberries
- ½ cup cold water
- 6 ice cubes
- 1/3 cup coconut milk
- 1/2 tsp vanilla powder
- 1 tsp erythritol
- 1 tsbp coconut oil

Preparation

1. Prepare the Ingredients by thoroughly washing and slicing the berries, removing ice cubes from the tray, and placing the water into the refrigerator until you are ready for it

2. Put all of the Ingredients into a blender. Make sure that the raspberries are on the bottom, followed by the ice cubes, the water, the coconut milk, the vanilla powder, the erythritol, and then the coconut oil

3. Blend on high until everything is smoothly mixed

4. Pour into a glass

5. Place a raspberry on top (if you wish) and enjoy

Pecan and Chocolate Bark

Time: 60 Minutes | Serves 10
Macros: Calories: 85 | Fats: 10g | Carbs: 1g |Protein: 2g

Ingredients

- ½ cup unsweetened cocoa powder
- 1 cup coconut oil
- 1/3 cup of some type of nut butter
- ¼ cup of non-sugar sweetener
- 1/2 tsp vanilla powder
- 1 tsp vanilla extract
- ½ cup unsweetened coconut flakes
- 1 tsp almond extract
- ½ tsp salt

Preparation

1. Line a small cookie sheet with wax paper, pressing down to ensure that the paper stays in place

2. Place the coconut oil and the nut butter in a pan on the stovetop. On low heat, melt them while stirring constantly. Once they are fully combined, move on to the next step

3. Mix in all of the additional Ingredients, one at a time.

4. When everything is combined, take the pan off of the stove

5. Pour the chocolate and nut butter mixture onto the cookie sheet. Put the cookie sheet immediately into the freezer

6. After 45 minutes, take the sheet out of the freezer. Use a sharp implement to break the chocolate bark into pieces.

Bonus! 10 Keto Diet Tips

Following the Keto diet requires some work. It's like any other diet in that you really need to focus on the foods that you eat. You may find yourself constantly reading the backs of packaging in order to determine how many carbs are in each serving. One thing that makes this easier is only eating whole foods. This way, you won't have to worry about that packaging – you just need to find items that are on the approved foods list or in your meal plans. There are several other things that you can do as well in order to ensure that you successfully follow the Keto diet. Here are ten of them.

Plan Out Your Meals in Advance

The better that you plan your meals, the more prepared you will be. It helps if you write out a schedule several days before the week starts, stating what you will be making and when. If you leave it up to chance, you might find yourself short an ingredient or reaching for a carb-laden snack. Advance planning keeps you from doing this.

Don't Keep Any Junk Food in theHouse

If you have junk food in your home, then you're more than likely going to find yourself reaching for it. You might also fall back on some bad habits. For example, if you regularly enjoyed snacks like cookies and brownies, and you happen to have some prepackaged onces present, then you might eat them in a moment of weakness. If you don't have those things present, then you obviously won't eat them.

Eat Snacks Throughout the Day

Although you'll feel much more full while you're on the Keto diet, you should still eat a snack and now and then. You'll feel better and it will keep your blood sugar on a much more even level. Look at it this way – if you are hungry in the time period between lunch and dinner and you don't have any Keto snacks on hand, you might reach for something that isn't diet-approved, like a (non-Keto) cookie. However, if you have a bag of almonds there and never reach that level of hunger, then you'll stay true to your diet.

Allow Yourself to Drink Caffeinated Beverages

Caffeine will help level out your moods and give you a nice boost when you're in the middle of a long workday. You don't need to cut out caffeine altogether in order to stay on the Keto diet. In fact, there's even a Keto approved coffee beverage called bulletproof coffee. (It's coffee with butter and heavy cream mixed in it, for the record.) As long as you don't add sugar to your coffee or tea, or fall for one of those fancy coffee house beverages, you'll be in good shape.

Breakfast Is the Most Important Meal of the Day

Breakfast is important no matter what, but it's especially crucial when you're on the Keto diet. Make sure to eat a healthy breakfast every morning, or if you run out of time, create a few smoothie mixes beforehand and throw them in the blender before you run out of the door. Breakfast is a crucial for those macros and micros, and to keep your stomach full.

Include Vegetables With Every Meal

The Keto diet might seem like a good excuse to eat nothing but meat all of the time. And while you do need to eat quite a bit of meat, you also need to balance it with other foods, like vegetables. Root vegetables are out, because they contain far too many carbs, but there are dozens of green vegetables that you can eat. Consider keeping some lettuce and spinach on hand and then throw together a salad with every meal.

Find Good Substitutes For Your Favorite Snacks

There are plenty of Keto-friendly substitutes for your favorite snacks out there. For example, if you like potato chips, which you can't have while on the Keto diet, grab a bag of pork rinds instead. Those have the same amount of crunch, but they're also something that you can eat without worrying about sending your body out of ketosis. Do a bit of research and find substitutes for the foods that you like the most.

Make Sure to Track Your Micros and Macros

You need to track your macros and micros every single day. They will help you ensure that you're receiving the right nutrients (it isn't about just eating bacon all of the time), and that you're not getting too many carbs and sugars in your diet. You need to eat properly Keto-balanced meals. Tracking these numbers will help.Seek Out Other Keto DietersIt always helps to have a support group on hand. Look on social media, such as Facebook, in order to see if you can find a group of Keto dieters. Then, join that group. It doesn't matter if they're local or not, as long as they can help you with your Keto diet journey. Your support group will be able answer questions and generally help you stay positive about the diet.

Remember That It's Mind Over Matter

Positive thinking is important. Those first few weeks on the Keto diet might be tough ones. If you end up thinking that it's impossible to follow the diet, then it will be! You need to think positively and know that you can do it. Once you've followed the diet for around a month or so, it will ingrained and you won't have to focus on it so much anymore. It does get easier!

Disclaimer

This book is intended to be informative and helpful and contains the opinions and ideas of the author. The author intends to teach in an entertaining manner. Some recipes may not suit all readers. Use this book and implement the guides and recipes at your own will, taking responsibility and risk where it falls. This work with all its contents, does not guarantee correctness, completion, quality or correctness of the provided information. Misinformation or misprints cannot be completely eliminated.

Imprint

Kylie Reid by proxy of:
Rocka Maldini
Roka Maldini
120, Old Railway Track
SVR 9017
Santa Venera
Malta
Malta
malta.publishing@gmail.com
Copyright 2019

Cover:
Design: Alima Media Turk

Printed in Great
Britain
by Amazon